Guide to Immunization Program Evaluation
for Grantees

November 2007

Acknowledgements

The Health Services Research and Evaluation Branch, Immunization Services Division would like to thank the following individuals for their contributions, guidance, and permission to utilize their programs' tools and resources. In particular, we would like to thank Maureen Wilce and the evaluation staff from the Division of Tuberculosis Elimination and the Division of Sexually Transmitted Diseases Prevention for allowing us to utilize their documents and templates. Without them, this guide would not be possible.

Faruque Ahmed
Betty Apt
Tom Chapel
Robin Curtis
Nancy Fasano
John Flynn
Paul Garrison
Holly Groom
Janet Kelly
Allison Kennedy
Maureen Kolasa
Megan Lindley
Suchita Lorick
James Lutz
Melinda Mailhot
Mark Messonnier
Bobby Babak Rasulnia
Richard Schieber
Michael Schooley
Carol Stanwyck
Shannon Stokley
John Stevenson
Maureen Wilce
Bayo Willis
Pascale Wortley

Table of Contents

Introduction: An overview of program evaluation

What is program evaluation?

Program evaluation is the systematic investigation of the structure, activities, or outcomes of public health programs. It explores whether activities are implemented as planned and outcomes have occurred as intended, and why. Evaluation provides grantees with the evidence they need to shape effective immunization programs by helping them to:

- Assess and improve existing programs
- Understand reasons for performance
- Plan and implement new programs
- Manage programs effectively
- Demonstrate the value of their efforts
- Ensure accountability

Evaluation can help support program implementation, and through its activities, builds on the program monitoring activities that immunization programs currently conduct in assessing whether program objectives (see Appendix A for a definition) have been met. For the first time
in 2008, immunization program grantees are required to engage in program evaluation activities. The Immunization Services Division has established three interrelated goals (see Appendix A for a definition) for grantee self-evaluation:

Goal 1: Immunization programs will have the skills needed to conduct ongoing evaluation to improve public health outcomes
Goal 2: Immunization programs will engage in program evaluation activities
Goal 3: Immunization programs will use evaluations to improve programs

Monitoring vs. Evaluation

Program monitoring is part of the evaluation process and provides a core data source on which to build a program evaluation. While monitoring tracks program outcomes, evaluation examines the factors that contribute to those outcomes. Evaluation activities should generally build on ongoing self-assessment activities and use data from these routine data collection processes.

We monitor our programs…but monitoring is not evaluation.

Program monitoring:
- Tracks outcomes, such as the 4:3:1:3:3:1 series coverage.
- Using an automotive analogy, monitoring is akin to keeping an eye on the warning lights on the dashboard of your car.

Program Evaluation:
- Systematically assesses the implementation and impact of programs, with the oal of understanding what contributes to program results.
- Helps programs answer the questions "What contributes to the success of my program?" and "How can I do better?"
- Involves looking under the hood to understand why the dashboard light is illuminated and to figure out what to do about it.

Vaccination coverage rates are the most frequently used indicators, but they are insufficient for understanding where we are on track and what direction are we going. At present, some program components have well-developed indicators, for example perinatal hepatitis B prevention, or IIS, while others do not. There is an effort underway to develop indicators across all program components.

Evaluation vs. Research

While there is some degree of overlap between evaluation and research, there are important differences between them. These differences, however, are often a matter of degree and are not necessarily "black and white" differences. The main purposes of **evaluation** are focused on identifying a specific program's achievements in meeting its goals and objectives, addressing program needs, identifying program operations, components, and activities that need to be improved, and solving practical problems. The main purposes of **research** are to create new knowledge in a field, knowledge that may be generalized to programs or populations throughout a field, and to test hypotheses.

Why conduct program evaluation?

Evaluation can benefit programs by allowing managers to direct scarce resources to those activities that move the program closer to national goals. This may also involve moving away from activities that do not help the program accomplish its mission (such as services that have been provided in the past but have little impact on progress toward objectives).

Reasons to conduct program evaluation include:

- Improving operations, achieving better outcomes, or achieving outcomes more efficiently
- Determining how well activities are being carried out and whether the activities are leading to the intended results
- Improving your own program, not to make generalizations about the impact of specific activities

Program evaluation should always be tailored to each program's unique circumstances. Each program can build on its strengths and design its own solutions, with evaluation acting as a catalyst for program improvement. There are many models for evaluation; no single option is right for every program. The evaluation approach and model will depend in part on the program's capacity and stage of development.

What is the CDC Framework for Program Evaluation?

CDC has developed an easy-to-use, well-researched framework for program evaluation (available at http://www.cdc.gov/eval/framework.htm) to help all types of public health programs systematically evaluate virtually any component. [1] The framework includes six steps (see below) and although presented sequentially, these evaluation steps often overlap. This Guide to Immunization Program Evaluation is based on the CDC's framework for evaluation. The Immunization Services Division recommends that immunization grantees use this Guide to organize and systematize their program evaluation activities.

CDC's Framework for Program Evaluation Steps:

1. Engage stakeholders
2. Describe the program
3. Focus the evaluation design
4. Gather credible evidence
5. Justify conclusions
6. Ensure use and share lessons learned

What's next?

Now that you're ready to start the evaluation process, use "Chapter 1: Getting Started with Program Evaluation" to learn more about how to form an evaluation team at your program and develop a plan to engage stakeholders. "Chapter 2: Guide to Writing an Immunization Program Evaluation Plan" will guide you through the six steps of the CDC Framework to help you construct your evaluation plan.

The evaluation plan lays the groundwork of design and preparation for the evaluation cycle outlined in the CDC's Framework for Program Evaluation. The evaluation plan, and the process of creating it, ensures the careful consideration of the potential uses and users of the evaluation, and how staff and stakeholders may react to its findings. Through its design, the evaluation solicits and incorporates feedback throughout the process to build support, avoid unpleasant surprises, and ensure the use of evaluation findings. Additional program evaluation resources can be found on the Immunization Program Evaluation Website at
http://www.cdc.gov/vaccines/programs/progeval/

---

[1] Centers for Disease Control and Prevention (CDC). 1999. "Framework for Program Evaluation in Public Health." Morbidity and Mortality Weekly Report 48(RR11):1-40.

Chapter 1: Getting started with program evaluation

> - This chapter provides the **five** preliminary actions that will enable grantees to get started with the program evaluation process.
>
> - Detailed, step-by-step guidance about how to engage stakeholders and plan your evaluation can be found in "Chapter 2: Writing an Immunization Program Evaluation Plan."

1. Identify a program component for evaluation

It is important to take the time to consider the many activities covered under your program in order to make a thoughtful and deliberate decision about what program component you want to evaluate. Some factors to consider in selecting the component:

- Where am I spending the most, in terms of time or funding?
- Where am I concerned the most, do we have known problem areas?
- Where are my big opportunities, what are some new program activities?
- Where are my big successes, what can we learn from successful efforts?

Based on these and other relevant factors, choose one of the ten priority immunization program components (listed below and in your IPOM available at http://www.cdc.gov/vaccines/vac-gen/policies/ipom/default.htm).

Immunization Program Components

Adolescent immunization	Population assessment
Adult immunization	Provider quality assurance
Education/training	Surveillance
Immunization information systems (IIS)	Vaccine accountability & management
Perinatal hepatitis B	Women Infants Children Program (WIC)

2. Form an evaluation team

The members of the program evaluation team will help design and/or conduct the evaluation. This team within your program may include people who have no prior knowledge of evaluation.

Listed below are some guidelines for building a multidisciplinary evaluation team:

- Build an evaluation team that encompasses epidemiological, data, and program practice skills related to the program component you have decided to evaluate (e.g. AFIX or adolescent immunization)
- Assign team roles and responsibilities

- Ensure the team has the time it needs to address evaluation activities (e.g., by setting aside regular meeting times)
- Provide team or individual training as needed

3. Designate an evaluation team lead

Designating one staff member as the evaluation team lead establishes a single point of contact for other staff and partners involved in evaluating the program. The evaluation team lead will enhance the visibility of evaluation efforts through collaborative planning and coordinated implementation. To ensure success, it is critical for program leadership to:

- Provide the evaluation team lead with appropriate time and resources
- Clarify responsibilities of the evaluation team lead
- Ensure authority of the evaluation team lead

The evaluation team lead's roles and responsibilities may include:

- Oversight of all evaluation activities
- Meeting coordinator for the evaluation team
- Principal analyst of the evaluation data
- Primary author of the evaluation plan or reports
- Point person for the dissemination of evaluation reports and materials

Once assembled, each team member's roles and responsibilities should be clearly defined. Remember, you will most likely make adjustments as the evaluation evolves. Table 1 below provides one example (see Appendix B for a sample table).

Table 1: Evaluation Team Roles and Responsibilities

Name and job title	Role	Responsibilities
Example: Jane Doe, Nurse, State AFIX Coordinator	*AFIX evaluation team leader*	*Provide input in drafting evaluation plan; Help collect and analyze data*

4. Assess the evaluation team's capabilities and resources to conduct an evaluation

Assessing the team's ability to conduct evaluations involves examining and understanding your program's evaluation related capabilities and resources. The assessment should consider:

- Program's commitment to evaluation
- Organizational culture and systems, both within and outside of the program
- Funding
- Staff time, knowledge, skills, and abilities
- Existing program evaluation tools and lessons learned

- Available data and information systems
- Potential barriers to evaluation
- Feasibility of strategies to address barriers

5. Evaluation team should identify (i.e. list) relevant stakeholders and conduct a stakeholder assessment

Stakeholders are people with vested interests in the program and who are potentially affected by evaluations. Stakeholders can be divided into four major categories (may not be mutually exclusive) shown in the table below.

Stakeholder Types	Definition	Examples
Decision makers	Decide and direct program operations, including how evaluation findings are used	Immunization program director, program manager, health department director, health commissioner, legislators
Implementers	Involved in program operations	Immunization program director, program manager, program staff, local public health staff
Participants	Served by the program	Physicians, parents, community members
Partners	Support/invested in immunization program or target population	Managed care plans, health systems, AAP and AAFP chapters, community-based organizations

Why should stakeholders be included from the beginning of the evaluation process?
- To reduce distrust and fear of evaluation
- To increase their awareness of and commitment to the evaluation process
- To increase the chances that stakeholders will adhere to subsequent recommendations that may affect their activities
- To increase the credibility of your evaluation findings

The level of involvement of stakeholders will vary depending on the component being evaluated, but priority stakeholders include those who can do one or more of the following:
- Increase the credibility of the evaluation efforts
- Will participate in the implementation of the program activities
- Will advocate or can authorize changes to the program based on findings of these evaluation activities
- Will fund or authorize improvements to the program.

There is no right or wrong number of stakeholders; the size and composition will likely depend on the component being evaluated and could change as the evaluation evolves. Keep in mind that larger groups will take longer to reach decisions and may make the process more complicated. Depending on the context and stage of development (see Chapter 2: pgs 14-15 for more details) of your program component, categories of stakeholders appropriate for engagement and their levels of involvement may vary widely. While you may already know your program stakeholders well, you will need to reconsider their perspectives in regard to program evaluation. For each stakeholder you have identified, consider:

- What is their interest in or perspective on the program and the evaluation?
- What is their role in the evaluation?
- How and when will they be engaged in the evaluation?

Often, the roles of stakeholders will change during an evaluation. You may need to revise your plan several times as changes occur. Table 2 below provides one example - see Appendix B for a sample table.

Table 2: Stakeholder assessment and engagement

Name and job title	Interest(s) or perspective(s) on evaluation	Role(s) in the evaluation	How and when to engage
Example: Jane Doe, AFIX field staff coordinator	Interested in continuous program improvement; evaluation directly impacts her day-to- day activities and the activities of her staff	Input on evaluation design, methods, and interpretation and use of results	Invite to initial stakeholder meeting, can provide technical assistance as needed throughout evaluation process; meet to review results of

What's next?

Now that you are prepared to engage and collaborate with your stakeholders, "Chapter 2: Writing an immunization program evaluation plan" will guide you through the six steps of the CDC Framework for Program Evaluation and help you develop and document an evaluation plan.

Remember, evaluation is a cyclical process, rather than a linear one. That is, successful evaluations lead to program improvements and suggest new areas for evaluation. Evaluation is not an end in itself but rather an approach to improving immunization programs.

In an era of limited resources, immunization programs may be concerned about funding evaluation activities and ensuring that these activities do not take away from other core program activities. It may take time to build staff capability and executive support for evaluation. Progress toward the evaluation goals outlined above may be incremental. CDC is committed to providing grantees with the training and technical assistance they need to successfully implement and sustain program evaluation activities. Additional program evaluation resources can be found on the Immunization Program Evaluation Website at http://www.cdc.gov/vaccines/programs/progeval/

Chapter 2: Writing an immunization evaluation plan

> This chapter provides detailed, step-by-step guidance about how to plan and write your program's evaluation plan.

Program Component

See Chapter 1 for information about choosing your evaluation component.

> *** To Do:**
> Your evaluation plan should specify the program component you have chosen.

Evaluation Goal(s)

Your evaluation plan should be guided by the goal(s) you are striving towards. A goal is a broad, overarching statement that explains why the evaluation is taking place. It (they) should be related to the component you have chosen to evaluate.

Examples:
- To determine the effectiveness of the program or program component
- To help equitably redistribute program resources
- To reduce rates of perinatal transmission of hepatitis B.
- To increase rates of adolescent vaccination.

> *** To Do:**
> Your evaluation plan should include the goal(s) related to the program component you have chosen.

Evaluation Team

See Chapter 1 for details about forming your evaluation team.

> *** To Do:**
> Your evaluation plan should include Table 1, "Evaluation Team Roles and Responsibilities" (Appendix B, page 34) **or** list and briefly describe each member's title, role and responsibilities.

Step 1: Engaging Stakeholders

> *In "Getting started", you identified relevant stakeholders for your program component and determined their expected level of involvement in the evaluation and at what point this involvement would begin. This section provides additional guidance on how to engage your stakeholders*

Tips: How to engage stakeholders?
Invite the stakeholders you have identified to a meeting, a conference call or series of meetings and calls, depending on how much time they have available to spend with you. In most cases, these are individuals with whom you already have working relationships. You can brief stakeholders on the program component that you want to evaluate, and obtain a clear understanding of stakeholder interests, perceptions, and concerns about your evaluation. You can also establish roles and responsibilities for stakeholders related to the evaluation and make sure that all internal and external stakeholders understand and agree to these tasks.

As discussed in "Getting started," there is no right or wrong number of stakeholders to include in your evaluation planning process; larger groups will take longer to reach decisions than smaller groups, and may make the process more complicated. One method that may be useful for gaining consensus among stakeholders is the Nominal Group Technique (NGT), which uses structured small-group discussion to generate and prioritize ideas from multiple stakeholders. For more information on the NGT, please see http://www.cdc.gov/HealthyYouth/evaluation/pdf/brief7.pdf

Involve stakeholders in key activities throughout the planning and implementation of the evaluation activities including describing your program component, developing and prioritizing evaluation questions, selecting appropriate evaluation methods, reviewing evaluation results and making recommendations, and disseminating evaluation findings.

Tips: How to maintain stakeholder engagement through the life of your program component evaluation?
- Maintain open, honest, and regular communication with the stakeholders by keeping them up to date on issues pertaining to the evaluation.
- Incorporate stakeholders' opinions and insights into the evaluation process.
- Identify during the initial meetings possible conflicts between stakeholders (e.g., competition, rivalry, and existing power structures) and facilitate productive working arrangements.
- Identify stakeholders' barriers to participation, and address them when possible.
- Plan before meeting or requesting assistance so that everyone's time can be spent wisely.
- Express gratitude and positive reinforcement verbally, and if possible, in more tangible ways (e.g., letter of appreciation, public recognition).
- Request volunteers for specific sub-tasks, if needed.

---

* To Do:
Your evaluation plan should include Table 2, "Stakeholder assessment and engagement" (Appendix C, page 35) **or** list and briefly describe each stakeholder including each person/group's: name, job title, interest/perspective, role, and how and when you engaged (or plan to engage) the stakeholder.

Step 2: Describing the Immunization Program Component

> *In "Getting started" you selected a program component to evaluate. The purpose of this section of the plan is to describe this component. <u>This description will ensure that all evaluation stakeholders have a shared understanding of your program component including its objectives, activities, and outcomes.</u> It will also identify any unfounded assumptions or logical gaps in your evaluation planning. Once completed, the program component description will lead naturally into your logic model.*

Background

The background for this program component can be addressed by considering the series of questions listed below. Remember, there are no "right" answers.

Example Questions:

- What problem does or should this program component address (e.g., ongoing perinatal transmission of hepatitis B, limited uptake of new adolescent vaccines, access to vaccine for low-income children)?
- What causes the problem (e.g., hospitals lacking standing orders for maternal HBsAg testing and birth dose administration, low rate of health care visits by 11-12 year-olds, cultural/language barriers)?
- What are the consequences of the problem (e.g., morbidity, costs, potential for outbreaks of vaccine-preventable disease, exclusion from school and day care)?
- What is the magnitude of the problem (e.g., potential for a large problem exists, but acting now may reduce this potential)?
- What changes or trends are occurring (e.g., pertussis incidence is increasing, demographic patterns are changing, decrease in completion of recommended vaccination series)?

Context

Context refers to the environment that affects your immunization program component's operations. Consider and explain the contextual factors in your evaluation plan as necessary.

These factors can include:

- How the immunization program collaborates and coordinates with other health and social services in the community, such as hospitals, schools, family planning clinics, and pharmacies.
- How the program component is funded – does it compete for resources with other public health programs within the community?
- Organization's structural factors (i.e., personnel, training, administrative regulations) that impact your program component's operations
- Policy and political environment surrounding your program component
- Community perceptions of vaccine-preventable disease

Stage of Program Development

Assessing the developmental stage of your program component will help you frame your evaluation and write your evaluation questions. The stage of development relates to how long the component's activities have been in existence and how long certain activities have been required.

The stage could be:
- Needs assessment
- Design and planning
- Implementation: early (e.g., less than a year) or middle?
- Well-established implementation (e.g., 13 years)

Stage of development will also help guide whether you might focus on evaluating processes, outcomes, or both (both are discussed in Step 3, page 19). For example, adolescent vaccination activities are largely in the early implementation phase, and therefore it is especially important to know how well program activities are being implemented. Preventing transmission of perinatal hepatitis B is in the well-established implementation phase, and therefore would lend itself to both process and outcome evaluation.

Target Population
The target population will again depend on your chosen component and could include one or more groups.

Examples:
- Parents of toddlers
- Adults and children without health insurance
- School-aged children and adolescents

Objectives
Your statement of objectives should refer back to your program component's goal(s). Objectives should be established that support this goal. Your program component's objectives are frequently national or state immunization objectives; however, your component may also have its own objectives. If your objectives are not established, it is an important part of your plan to do this now. (See appendix A).

If you plan to evaluate a program area that is not specifically addressed in your 2008 grant application and therefore one for which no SMART objectives have already been written, be sure the objectives you write are "**SMART**": **S**pecific, **M**easurable, **A**chievable, **R**elevant, and **T**ime-bound. Detailed explanations and examples of SMART objectives can be found in Appendix A.

Examples:
1. For a program that chose **adolescent vaccination**:

Goal	*Increase rates of adolescent vaccination.*
Objectives	1. *Increase the number of adolescent VFC providers from X to Y by January 2009.* 2. *Increase the proportion of adolescent vaccine providers who participate in the state immunization information system from 10% to 40% by Fall 2009.* 3. *Increase parental awareness around adolescent vaccination from 50% to 100% by January 2009.*

2. For a program that chose **preventing perinatal transmission of hepatitis B:**

Goal	*Reduce rates of perinatal transmission of hepatitis B.*
Objectives	1. *Increase the percent of hospitals that routinely administer the hepatitis B birth dose from 65% to 85% by January 2009.* 2. *Increase the percent of hospitals that have written standing orders for maternal HBsAg verification and testing on admission from 80% to 100% by January 2009.* 3. *Increase the percent of hospitals educated on new ACIP childhood hepatitis B recommendations related to perinatal transmission from 85% to 100% by January 2009.*

In addition to the above, different parts of a program component can be categorized into inputs, activities, outputs and outcomes. Definitions and examples are provided below. Table 3, "Program Component Description" (Appendix D) is provided for your use.

Inputs

Inputs are the resources that go into your program component (e.g., money, staff, and materials).

Examples:
- Immunization program staff
- 317 or VFC funding
- Infrastructure resources that are part of the health department
- Partner organizations

Activities

Activities are the actual events that take place as part of your program component.

Examples:
- Hiring and training new staff
- Policy development or revision
- Providing targeted outreach efforts for specific high-risk populations
- Educating patients, providers or community members
- Surveillance

Activities can be grouped as initial and subsequent activities. Although most activities in immunization programs are ongoing, some activities may need to be done before others. For example, conducting an AFIX office visit to assess coverage would occur before providing feedback to that office.

Outputs
Outputs are the direct products of the program component's activities.

Examples:
- A strategic plan for your program component
- The number of flu shot clinics held
- The number of providers educated about new vaccines for adolescents

Outputs are assessed to "show" that the program component is being implemented as planned. However, they are not indications of effectiveness. For example, we can record that 10 educational sessions were conducted but there's no direct indication whether people have learned or acted on their new knowledge about immunization. In short, outputs show what work was done, but do not indicate that changes have taken place or resulted due to these actions.

To identify your program component's outputs, consider each activity you listed in Table 3 and list corresponding outputs in the column to the right of your activities. For example, the output "providers educated about new vaccines for adolescents" corresponds to the activity, "educating patients, providers, or community members." The activity, "providing targeted vaccination clinics" corresponds to the output, "flu shot clinics held".

Outcomes
Outcomes are the **intended effects** of the program component's activities. They may or may not have been achieved. They are the changes you want to occur in patients, providers, or the community because of your program activities. These are typically thought of as short-, mid-, or long-term outcomes and should be tied to your program component objectives. Short-term outcomes are the immediate effects of your program component (e.g., changes in knowledge, attitudes, skills, awareness, or beliefs of the target population). Mid-term outcomes are intended effects of your program component that take longer to occur (e.g., changes in policy or individuals' behavior). Long-term outcomes are intended effects of your program component that may take several years to achieve.

Examples:
- Parents' knowledge is increased (short-term)
- Increased parental demand for vaccination (mid-term)
- Increased vaccination rates (long-term)

Some of the important changes we want to occur, however, are less direct or difficult to measure. Examples:
- Trust built within the community
- Parents seeking out recommended vaccines for themselves and loved ones

For these outcomes, "proxy" or indirect measures can be used to assess whether they have been achieved. Often, program staff may be able to suggest ways to measure these effects. For example, an outreach worker may "know" trust is built when a community member approaches him with a question about immunizations. These types of information can be incorporated and used in the evaluation. To identify your program component outcomes, consider the activities and outputs you listed in Table 3 and list corresponding outcomes in the column to the right.

Logic Model

A logic model is a graphic depiction of the program component. In other words, a logic model illustrates the logical links between the activities your program conducts and the outcomes you intend to achieve. An AFIX Logic Model is provided as an example in Figure 1 (Appendix E). Drawing a logic model during the evaluation planning process is important to define the associations among program resources, activities, and results.

For the evaluation, a logic model provides:
- A sense of scope – what are the elements of the program components? How are they interconnected?
- A "map" to help ensure that systematic decisions are made about what is to be measured in the evaluation process and to identify areas where clarification may be needed
- A framework for organizing indicators and for ensuring that none are overlooked

Using the resources, activities, outputs, and outcomes identified in the project description (Table 3), you can choose to develop a logic model for your program component. There are no "right" or "wrong" logic models, but the logic model must clearly show the complete paths linking inputs and activities to outcomes. You will probably need to review and revise your logic model many times throughout the evaluation. Logic models for selected program components and activities are being developed and will be posted on the Immunization Program Evaluation website at http://www.cdc.gov/vaccines/programs/progeval/ when completed. It may be useful to review these models prior to developing your own to see if one of these logic models can be used to describe your program component (with minor modifications).

---

* To Do:

Your evaluation plan should briefly describe the component including the following sections: background, context, stage of development, target population and list the objective(s) of your evaluation. Additionally, you should include Table 3, "Program Description" (Appendix D, page 36) **or** you can provide a list of each of the following: inputs, activities, outputs, outcomes. **Optional:** Attach the program component's logic model

---

Step 3: Focusing the Evaluation

> ➢ *Although the logic model depicting a program component may inspire many evaluation questions, it may not be feasible or useful to evaluate every element or path in your logic model. Thus, focusing your evaluation and selecting your evaluation questions are important steps. Focus will also ensure that the evaluation meets the needs of stakeholders and that the findings will be used as intended.*

Utility and Feasibility

Two important standards to keep in mind when focusing your evaluation are **utility** and **feasibility**. Your answers to the following questions will help you focus your evaluation by identifying what your stakeholders need to learn from the evaluation – the evaluation questions.

To maximize the **utility** of the evaluation, ask the following questions:
- Who will use the evaluation findings?
- How will the findings be used?
- What do they need to learn from the evaluation?

Table 4 below includes sample answers to the questions – your answers may vary depending on your chosen component. See appendix F for a sample table.

Table 4: Focusing the Evaluation Worksheet

Who will use the evaluation findings?	What do they need to learn from the evaluation?	How will the findings be used?
CDC	• Is the program component being implemented as designed? • Is the program component meeting its objectives? • What are the problem areas in implementing the program component?	• Justify that immunization program resources are being appropriately used.
Immunization program manager and staff		• Identify the extent to which program component was implemented. • Make midcourse adjustments to improve the program component's effectiveness. •
State/county HD staff	• Does program staff have knowledge and resources to achieve program component goals? •	• Modify/implement staff training
State/county legislators or policymakers	• Is the program component effective? • Are state/local funds for the program component being well used?	• Determine future funding level for the program component
Community-based organization (CBO) partners	• Are outreach efforts reaching the target population for the program component?	• Advocate for the program component in the community

Evaluation Questions

There are two basic types of evaluation questions:

Process questions focus on examining the implementation of the program component and determining whether activities are being implemented as planned and whether inputs and resources are being used effectively.

Outcome evaluation focuses on showing whether or not a program component is achieving the desired changes in patients, providers, or the community. Using your assessment of who will use the findings and how the findings will be used, identify key evaluation questions based on your program component description. Sample evaluation questions are shown below.

Examples:

Process questions:
1. Are there sufficient resources to carry out the activities of the selected program component?
2. Are providers receiving educational materials about new vaccines and recommendations?
3. Have community partners been engaged to collaborate with us to increase vaccine coverage in hard-to-reach populations?
4. Is AFIX staff appropriately trained?
5. Do hospitals have written protocols on perinatal hepatitis B prevention?
6. Are outreach efforts reaching the target population?

Outcome questions:
1. Do providers who receive AFIX visits make recommended changes?
2. Are providers routinely entering data into the IIS?
3. Is there an increase in awareness of the pneumococcal vaccine recommendation among high risk persons?
4. Did influenza vaccination rates increase in African Americans 65 years and older?
5. To what degree was the outreach effort able to increase completion of the 4:3:1:3:3:1 series?

The above questions illustrate potential questions covering a range of program components and activities. For any given component, you can generate a long list of questions. From your list, with consideration of **utility, feasibility, and the ability to produce accurate findings,** you will need to select a few (~3-5) high priority evaluation questions. Use the tips listed below to help you choose a few priority questions which should ideally include both processes and outcomes.

Tips: Prioritizing Evaluation Questions Based on Program and Stakeholders' Needs and Resources
- As with all the other steps, involve key stakeholders
- Brainstorm a list of evaluation questions about your chosen component
- Group your evaluation questions by theme
- Prioritize evaluation questions by applying the evaluation question criteria to your list of questions. Criteria include whether the question:
    o Is important to your program staff and stakeholders
    o Reflects key goals and objectives of your program
    o Reflects key elements of your program logic model
    o Will provide information you can act upon to make program improvements
    o Can be answered using available resources (e.g., time, budget, personnel)
    o Will be supported (in terms of resources needed to answer the question) by the program
    o Available data sources (What data do you already have or are already collecting for another purpose that may be useful for the evaluation? What data do you need?)
- Examine and categorize the prioritized list of questions as process or outcome evaluation questions.
- Relate your process evaluation questions to the process sections of your logic model (i.e., inputs, activities, outputs) and your outcome evaluation questions to the outcome sections of your logic model (i.e., short-term, intermediate, long-term outcomes).

Now, based on these few high priority questions, you need to choose an evaluation design and data collection methods (discussed in the next framework step).

Evaluation Design

Although program evaluation questions are geared to answering specific questions for specific program components, the designs for answering them often resemble research designs. However, it is important to remember that the purpose of evaluation is to **improve programs**, not to publish generalizable findings in a peer-reviewed journal, and therefore you need only collect data sufficient to answer your evaluation questions.

Key issues to consider about evaluation design:
- Will you have a control or comparison group?
- Will you measure before and after or only after?
- Will you collect data prospectively or retrospectively?
- Do you need in-depth, detailed information about the question(s) (qualitative information), or specific, targeted information (quantitative information)?

Additional considerations which are helpful in **selecting your design**:
- Standards of "good" evaluation. You will want to select a design that provides useful information to improve the immunization program component, and is not overly disruptive of daily operations. In addition, the design that is selected should produce accurate findings given the resources available for the evaluation.

- Timeliness. When do decisions need to be made about the program component?
- Stage of development. For a newly developed component, process evaluation helps us understand what we need to do in order to enhance the program component. In a well established program component, the addition of outcome evaluation may serve to help identify the component's performance and effectiveness.

---

* To Do:
See next step.

Step 4: Gathering Credible Evidence: Data Collection

> *This section provides information about how to gather the information you will need to help answer the evaluation questions you identified in the previous step. It includes the indicators you will use to determine program component success, benchmarks that will serve as targets to measure performance against, data collection methods and tools, and a timeline for data collection activities.*

Indicators

Indicators are measurable signs of a program component's performance. Good indicators are relevant, understandable, and useful. Indicators are tied to the objectives identified in the program description, the logic model and/or the evaluation questions. Some immunization program components, such as registries (IIS) and perinatal hepatitis B prevention, already have defined **indicators (also known as performance measures)** that can be found in the IPOM (see Appendix G for an abbreviated list). Note that these are a mix of process indicators that measure implementation activities as well as outcome indicators. An effort is underway to develop indicators for every program component and these will be made available once created. In the meantime, you may choose to write your own indicators if the program component you choose to evaluate does not have indicators specified by CDC. If you choose to write your own indicators, tie your indicators to a "SMART" objective as shown in the example below in Table 5 (see Appendix H for a sample table).

Guide to Immunization Program Evaluation for Grantees

Table 5: Objectives and Indicators Worksheet

Example:

Objective	Increase percentage of children entering kindergarten who completed 4:3:1:3:3:1: vaccination series from 80% to 90% by 2009.						
		VERB	METRIC	POPULATION	OBJECT	BASELINE MEASURE	GOAL MEASURE	TIMEFRAME
Breakdown		Increase	Percent	Children entering kindergarten	Completion of 4:3:1:3:3:1 series	80%	90%	By September 2009

	VERB	METRIC	POPULATIO	OBJECT	BASELINE MEASURE	GOAL MEASURE	TIMEFRAME
Breakdown	Increase	Percent	Children entering kindergarten	Completion of 4:3:1:3:3:1 series	80%	90%	By 2009
Indicator	Percent of children entering kindergarten in 2009 who had completed the 4:3:1:3:3:1 series.						

When your evaluation questions do not draw on existing program objectives, a strategy similar to that of the above worksheet can be used to develop indicators. Keeping in mind that indicators are visible and measurable signs of change identify some related, observable manifestations, using proxy measures as appropriate, making sure they are "SMART." Note that it is likely that you will have multiple indicators tied to each evaluation question. The table below provides some example indicators.

Evaluation Question	Possible manifestations...	Indicators
Example: Are underserved adults being reached with recommended vaccines?	*Uninsured adults who receive recommended vaccines*	*Percent of uninsured adult patients who received recommended vaccines.*
	Whether or not program resources are specifically devoted to adult immunization may indicate whether underserved adults are being targeted and reached	*Number of program FTEs focused on adult immunization*
	Forms and signs accessible to the low literate may indicate the effort to communicate with underserved adults	*Percent of signs and forms written for persons with low literacy levels*

Targets

Program targets are what the stakeholders of the immunization programs consider to be "reasonable expectations" for the program. In thinking about the program targets, it is important to think about what "success" means. How do you measure success? What does it mean if the program component is successful or effective? These standards that programs have set for themselves will be used as the benchmark against which you will measure your program component's performance. Targets may not exist that relate to all of your evaluation questions, but many standards are implicit in a program component's strategic plans. Stakeholders can also help you set standards. The example below (Table 6) illustrates how evaluation questions, indicators, and program targets relate to one another. See Appendix I for a sample table.

Table 6: Questions, Indicators and Targets Worksheet

Evaluation Question	Process and Outcome	Targets
Example: Are underserved adults being reached with recommended vaccines?	*Percent of uninsured adult patients who received recommended vaccines.*	*80% of uninsured adult patients received recommended vaccines*
	Number of program FTEs focused on adult immunization	*At least 0.5 program FTEs devoted to adult immunization*
	Percent of signs and forms written for persons with low-literacy levels	*All patient education signs and forms are written at a 6th grade reading level*

Data Collection

Your plan should include details about the "who", "what", "when" and "how" related to collecting the necessary data for each indicator. You can use Table 7 (Appendix J) as a worksheet to help describe your data collection plan.

Consider the following questions for each indicator:

- What methods will you use to collect the data?
- Where are the data?
- How often will it be collected?
- Who is responsible for collecting the data?
- How will you handle and store the data?
- How will you assure the accuracy of the data?

Data sources

Note that more than one data source may provide information for each indicator.

Examples:

- Records or charts
- Immunization information systems and other databases
- Interviews or focus groups
- Participant observations

Tools
Tools are the documents (e.g. questionnaires) or strategies (e.g. focus groups) you will use to collect the data you need. When choosing tools, consider whether the questions you are asking or data elements you are collecting are tied to your indicators.

Be sure to:
- Collect only the information you need
- Collect the information you need in the most straightforward way possible
- Use tools that are easy to understand and use, and do not place undue burdens on staff
- Pilot test tools to ensure that users can successfully use the tool for its intended purpose; make changes based on your pilot test

Human Subjects Consideration
At this point it is important to consider if your evaluation will require review by your program's Institutional Review Board (IRB). Many program evaluations are exempt from review but this is a consideration when developing your plan.

---

* To Do:
See next step.

Step 5: Justifying Conclusions: Analysis and Interpretation

> ➢ *This section provides information about considerations related to analyzing and interpreting the data you plan to collect.*

Analysis

Your data collection methods will guide the analysis plan. Although your initial analysis plan may be general, you may want to address issues such as:

- What data aggregation systems or software you plan to use
- What statistical methods (if any) you plan to use
- What stratifications (if any) you plan to examine among the data
- What types of tables or figures you may use

Tips: Analyzing the Evaluation Data
- Address data management issues to ensure uniformity in data handling
    - o If needed, transfer data from complex data collection tools to forms for data entry or transcribe data from field notes or audiotapes.
    - o Determine how you will code your data.
    - o Monitor data entry to ensure accuracy.

- Develop a data analysis plan
    - o Determine what analyses (quantitative and/or qualitative) need to be performed for each indicator.
    - o Modify your evaluation plan to include your plans for data analysis.

- Analyze your quantitative data
    - o Tabulate the data relevant to each indicator.
    - o If appropriate, make comparisons between groups to show differences and commonalties.
    - o Investigate change in your indicators over time.

- Analyze your qualitative data
    - o Read the qualitative data and identify similar responses/ideas.
    - o Mark and sort the qualitative data by themes/categories.

Table 8 below combines the outputs of this and the previous 2 steps of the framework – evaluation questions, indicators, targets, data collection and analysis. One example is provided below. See Appendix K for a sample table.

Example:

Table 8: Data Collection and Analysis

INDICATOR(S)	TARGET(S)	DATA SOURCE(S)	DATA COLLECTION	ANALYSIS
Evaluation Question: To what degree did the new parent outreach effort increase completion of the 4:3:1:3:3:1 series?				
Percent of children entering kindergarten in 2008 who completed the 4:3:1:3:3:1 series	*90% of children entering kindergarten in 2008 have completed the 4:3:1:3:3:1 series*	• *Charts or school immunization records* • *State immunization registry*	***Method:*** *Review charts and/or records* ***Timeline:*** *October-November 2008* ***Persons Responsible:*** *School nurses at all 42 kindergartens in state; state registry coordinator*	***Method:*** *Calculate percentages and frequencies with statistical software and compare to 2007 data* ***Timeline:*** *Complete by December 2008* ***Persons Responsible:*** *Immunization program statistician; project manager*

<u>Interpretation</u>
In this phase you will judge your findings against the program standards. In drawing conclusions from the evaluation findings, it is important to consider the context in which the program component is operating. It is also important that conclusions be sound, reasonable and objective. Involving the stakeholders in this process will bring insights and explanation to the evaluation findings, thus ensuring the validity of the interpretation and that recommendations based on the findings are relevant. Developing a draft report and sharing it with stakeholders is one method of involving stakeholders in the interpretation process and may be sufficient and appropriate in some cases.

Tips: Determine what the evaluation findings say about your program
- Organize your evaluation findings.
- Consider issues of context when interpreting the results.
- Determine the practical significance of what has been learned.
- Discuss what is working well and what is not.
- Discuss the limitations of the evaluation.
- Synthesize the evaluation findings.

---

* To Do:

Your evaluation plan should include Table 8, "Data Collection and Analysis" (Appendix K, page 43) **or** list and briefly describe the following: evaluation questions, the related indicators and targets, the data sources and methods and when and by whom data will be collected and analyzed.

Step 6: Ensuring Use and Sharing Lessons Learned: Reporting and Dissemination

> ➢ *A reporting and dissemination plan will ensure that evaluation findings will be distributed to those who will make use of the lessons learned from the evaluation. The plan should describe what medium you will use to disseminate the evaluation findings, who is responsible for disseminating the findings, how the findings will be used and who will act on the findings. The purpose of program evaluation is to use the information from the evaluation to improve program component operation and enhance its performance. <u>An evaluation does not achieve its purpose if it is not used!</u>*

In writing this section of your plan, check the reporting and dissemination plan against the stakeholder list and assessment you developed earlier (Table 2) to ensure that your reports will address stakeholder needs and that the reports will reach them.

Table 9 below provides one example (see Appendix L for a sample table).

Table 9: Disseminating Findings

PERSON/GROUP NAME	EVALUATION USES	DISSEMINATION METHODS
Example: State/county health department legislators or policymakers	*Determine future funding level for the program component*	*Full written report after evaluation is completed; Brief testimony before state Committee on Health and Social Services*

<u>Ensuring Use</u>
Throughout the evaluation process you will want to develop mechanisms to ensure that findings are used and changes implemented. Your plan should address how you plan to use your findings, in at least a general way. It may be appropriate to share findings with the public through different media outlets such as in a local newspaper or through public service announcements. Findings can also be shared with other grantees to increase awareness of identified opportunities. You will add to the list of uses as your evaluation progresses.

Tips: Ensuring effective evaluation reports
- Provide interim and final reports to intended users in time for use
- Tailor the report content, format, and style for the audience(s) by involving audience members
- Include a summary
- Summarize the description of the stakeholders and how they were engaged
- Describe essential features of the program (e.g., including logic models)
- Explain the focus of the evaluation and its limitations
- Include an adequate summary of the evaluation plan and procedures
- Provide all necessary technical information (e.g., in appendices)
- Specify the standards and criteria for evaluative judgments
- Explain the evaluative judgments and how they are supported by the evidence

- List both strengths and weaknesses of the evaluation
- Discuss recommendations for action with advantages, disadvantages, and resource implications
- Ensure protections for program clients and other stakeholders
- Anticipate how people or organizations might be affected by the findings
- Present minority opinions or rejoinders where necessary
- Verify that the report is accurate and unbiased
- Organize the report logically and include appropriate details
- Remove technical jargon
- Use examples, illustrations, graphics, and stories

---

* To Do:

Your evaluation plan should include Table 9, "Disseminating Findings" (Appendix L, page 44) **or** briefly describe with whom you will share the findings of the evaluation, how these findings will be useful to them and what methods (and format) you will use to share these findings.

What's next?

Submit your evaluation plan in August 2008 as part of the 2009 grant application. The Immunization Services Division will provide feedback on these plans and further guidance about requirements (e.g. progress reports) for future grant applications.

Now that you have developed an evaluation plan, you and your stakeholders are ready to enter the next phase – conducting your evaluation! The time required to conduct your evaluation will vary depending on the complexity and focus of your evaluation. Once the evaluation is completed, some programs may elect to implement changes based on the findings of the evaluation and evaluate the effectiveness of these changes, others may undertake an evaluation of a different program component.

Please visit the Immunization Program Evaluation website at http://www.cdc.gov/vaccines/programs/progeval/ for updates and additional resources. If you have any questions or concerns related to this evaluation please contact your project officer or email the Immunization Services Division evaluation workgroup (email address will be posted on the Immunization Program Evaluation website).

Appendix A
Goals and Objectives

WHAT IS A GOAL?

A broad statement of program purpose that describes the expected long-term effects of a program.

WHAT IS AN OBJECTIVE?

Your program objectives are statements describing the results to be achieved and the manner in which they will be achieved. Objectives are more immediate than goals; they are the mileposts you will pass on the way to achieving your program goal(s). Because objectives detail your program activities, you usually need multiple objectives to address a single goal. Well-written and clearly defined objectives will help you monitor your progress toward achieving your program goals and set targets for accountability.

HOW CAN YOU WRITE AN OBJECTIVE THE "SMART" WAY?

Your objectives will be appropriate and effective if you follow the SMART technique for writing objectives. The attributes of a SMART objective are: Specific, Measurable, Achievable, Relevant, and Time-bound.

Specific

Making your objectives specific means including the "who," "what," and "where" of the objective. "Who" refers to your target population (e.g., school-aged children). "What" refers to the action (e.g., vaccinate, identify). "Where" refers to the location of the action (e.g., public health clinic in City X). Be as specific as possible about the target population (e.g., male and female adolescents between the ages of 15-19 years, instead of "adolescents").

When describing the action, use only one action verb per activity (e.g., develop a workshop instead of develop and implement a workshop). More than one verb means that more than one action must be measured, which will cause problems when it comes to measuring success.

Also, avoid verbs with vague meanings (e.g., "understand", "do") when describing expected results. Instead, use verbs that reflect measurable action, such as "identify" or "list".

Remember: The greater the specificity, the greater the possibility for measurement.

Measurable

Your objectives need to be measurable. Here the focus is on "how much" change is expected. Your objectives should quantify the amount of change you hope to achieve (e.g., Project area X will implement 2 professional development workshops among all immunization providers in City X by January 2009.). "2" and "all" represent the "how much" of the objective.

Achievable

Your objectives should be realistic given your program resources and planned implementation. For instance, if you read the following: "100% of women in project area X will be vaccinated against hepatitis A" you realize that this is not achievable. Besides the fact that reaching 100% of women is unrealistic, you will be wasting resources because not all women are at risk for hepatitis A. You can use state, county, or local statistics as well as data from similar immunization programs to provide context for what is reasonable and to help you ensure that your program objectives are achievable.

Relevant

Objectives are relevant when they relate directly to the program's goals and together represent reasonable programmatic steps that can be implemented within a specific timeframe. For instance, a program goal is "Reduce neonatal hepatitis B in City X". A relevant objective may be: "By December 2008, increase the percentage of women (from X% to Y%) in City X receiving a test for hepatitis B surface antigen at first prenatal visit."

Time-bound

Your objectives should be defined within a timeframe. Here the focus is on "when" the objective will be met. Specifying a timeframe in the objective will help you in both planning and evaluating your program (e.g., by January 2009).

PROCESS VS. OUTCOME OBJECTIVES

You can write two types of objectives: process and outcome. When you write a process objective, you describe the activities/services that will be delivered as part of implementing the program. When you write an outcome objective, you specify the intended effect of the program in the target population or end result of a program. The outcome objective focuses on what your target population(s) will know or will be able to do at the conclusion of your program/activity.

SHORT-TERM, MID-TERM, AND LONG-TERM OUTCOME OBJECTIVES

You can categorize outcome objectives as short-term, mid-term, or long-term. They should be logically linked to each other and to the process objectives.

- Short-term outcome objectives are the initial expected changes in your target population(s) after implementing certain activities or interventions (e.g., changes in knowledge, skills, and attitudes).

- Mid-term outcome objectives are those interim results that provide a sense of progress toward reaching the long-term objectives (e.g., changes in behavior, norms, and policy).

- Long-term outcome objectives are achieved only after the program has been in place for some time (e.g., changes in mortality, morbidity, quality of life).

Guide to Immunization Program Evaluation for Grantees

Appendix B

Table 1: Evaluation Team Roles and Responsibilities

Name and job title	Role	Responsibilities

Appendix C

Table 2: Stakeholder Assessment and Engagement

Name and job title	Interest(s) or perspective(s) on evaluation	Role(s) in the evaluation	How and when to engage

Appendix D

Table 3: Program Component Description

Inputs	Activities		Outputs	Outcomes	
	Initial	Subsequent		Short-/Mid-term	Long-term

Appendix E
Figure 1: AFIX Logic Model

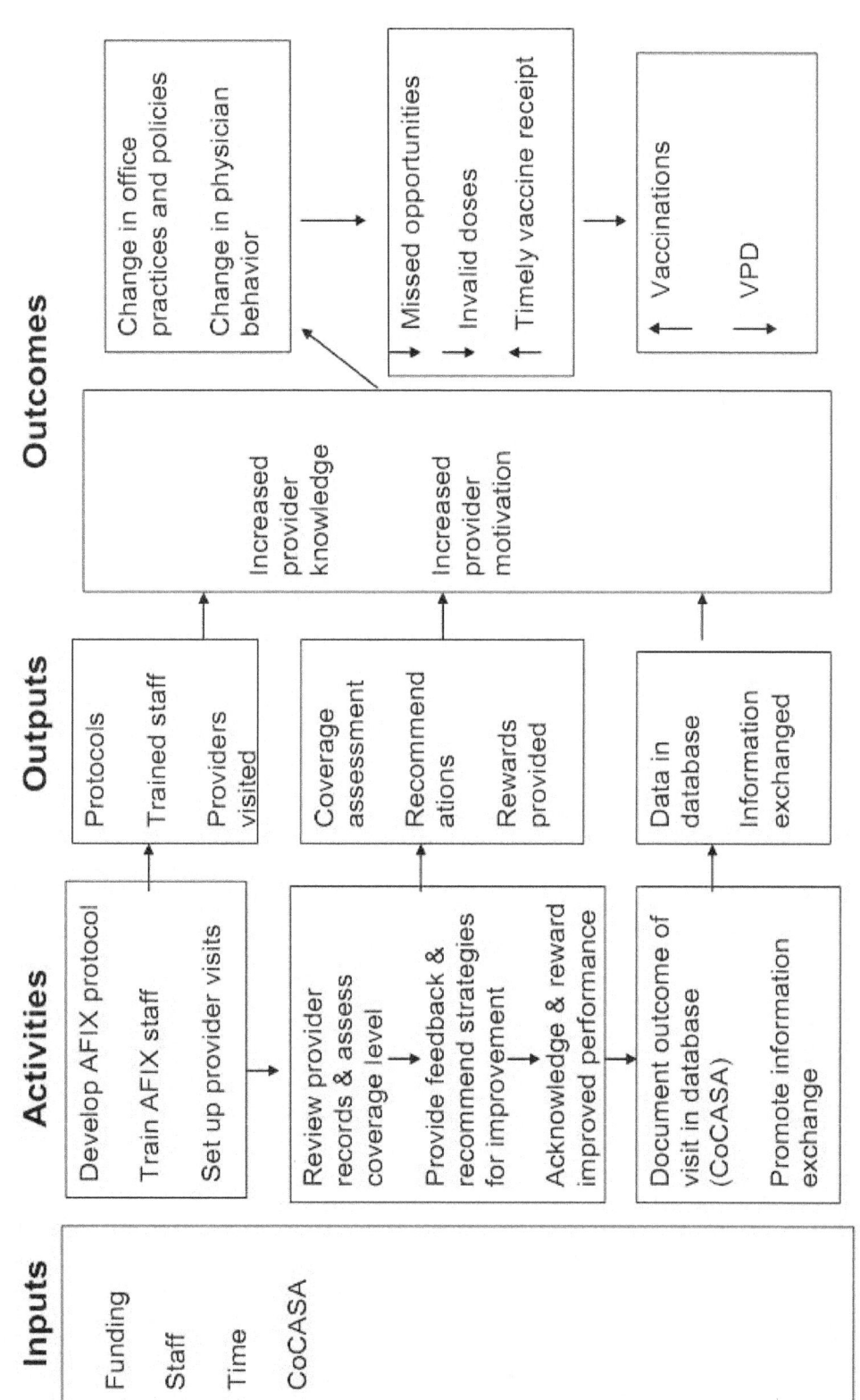

Guide to Immunization Program Evaluation for Grantees

Appendix F

Table 4: Focusing the Evaluation Worksheet

Who will use the evaluation findings?	What do they need to learn from the evaluation?	How will the findings be used?

Appendix G

Examples of Immunization Program Component Indicators

Below are selected indicators for some of the immunization program components listed in the IPOM. Please note that not all program components or indicators are included in this Appendix.

IIS
- Proportion of children <6 in IIS catchment area who are participating in IIS
- Proportion of immunization coverage for children 19-35 months of age and children <6 years of age in the IIS catchment area who are participating in the IIS
- Number and proportion of private provider sites submitting immunization events to the IIS on children <6 years of age.

Perinatal Hepatitis B
- Percentage of delivery hospitals with a) written policies and procedures, and b) written standing orders for maternal HBsAg verification and testing (when appropriate) on admission for delivery.
- Proportion of infants born to HBsAg-positive mothers who complete their vaccination series by 6-8 months of age if the infant is received single antigen or Pediarix vaccine and by 15 months if the infant received the Comvax vaccine series
- Proportion of identified household and sexual contacts for which susceptibility status is determined.

Education, information, training, and partnerships
- Proportion of providers who are given directions to subscribe to the automatic notification of new VISs, and number who actually subscribe to the updates
- Number of events planned within the state entered into the NIIW database
- Number of PSA or NIIW materials that were utilized or distributed

Epidemiology and surveillance
- Proportion of case reports submitted to CDC within one month of diagnosis
- Proportion of Hib cases among children <5 with complete vaccination history
- Proportion of probable and confirmed pertussis cases meeting the clinical case definition that is laboratory confirmed

Population Assessment
- Percentage of children, adolescents, non-institutionalized adults, or institutionalized adults who have received specific vaccines or vaccine series, as specified by Healthy People 2010 objectives.
- Percentage of children entering school who have received all recommended vaccines
- Percentage of child care facility enrollees who are age-appropriately immunized

Appendix H
Table 5: Objectives and Indicators Worksheet

Objective		VERB	METRIC	POPULATION	OBJECT	BASELINE MEASURE	GOAL MEASURE	TIMEFRAME
Breakdown								

		VERB	METRIC	POPULATION	OBJECT	BASELINE MEASURE	GOAL MEASURE	TIMEFRAME
Breakdown								
Indicator or Performance measure								

41

Guide to Immunization Program Evaluation for Grantees

Appendix I

Table 6: Questions, Indicators and Targets Worksheet

Evaluation Question	Process and Outcome Indicators	Targets

Guide to Immunization Program Evaluation for Grantees

Appendix J

Table 7: Data Collection Worksheet

Indicator	Data Sources	Collection		
		Who	When	How

Guide to Immunization Program Evaluation for Grantees

Appendix K

Table 8: Data Collection and Analysis

INDICATOR(S)	TARGET(S)	DATA SOURCE(S)	DATA COLLECTION	ANALYSIS
Evaluation Question:				
			Method: Timeline: Person Responsible:	Method: Timeline: Person Responsible:
Evaluation Question:				
			Method: Timeline: Person Responsible:	Method: Timeline: Person Responsible:
Evaluation Question:				
			Method: Timeline: Person Responsible:	Method: Timeline: Person Responsible:

Appendix L

Table 9: Disseminating Findings

PERSON/GROUP NAME	EVALUATION USES	DISSEMINATION METHODS

Guide to Immunization Program Evaluation for Grantees

This document can be found on the CDC website at:
http://www.cdc.gov/vaccines/programs/progeval/downloads/ipe_guide_11-2007.pdf

www.ingramcontent.com/pod-product-compliance
Lightning Source LLC
Chambersburg PA
CBHW081800170526
45167CB00008B/3259